The Science of Growing Hair in the Year 2020:
Grow, Keep and Boost It Now
Melissa Toyos, MD

To my husband who inspires and supports me in every way, the girls who are my reason in this life, and my Toyos Clinic family. And lastly, to Auge the opinionated, misbehaved dachschund who completes our family.

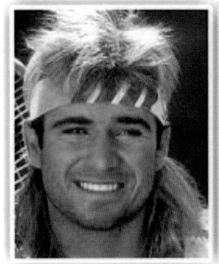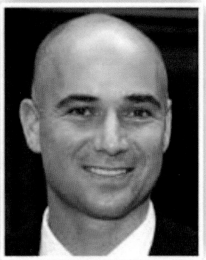

Losing my hair was like losing "little pieces of my identity."

\- *Andre Agassi*

Table of Contents:

Getting Into Hair

Attending a hair transplant conference, I did a quick scan of the room. The hair transplant surgeons at this meeting were overwhelmingly male, most of them had personal experience with hair loss and transplant surgeries, sometimes just one surgery, sometimes four or more but with full heads of hair to show for it. Some of them were sporting mullets, just because they could, I guess. Full, dramatic hair was good advertising. The surgeons were from every specialty too: the dermatologists that you expect here and there but also general surgeons, nephrologists, ear nose and throat doctors. I did not, however, run into one ophthalmologist. So how did an eye surgeon get started in hair restoration? I've spent over twenty years focusing on one tiny organ and on microsurgery to correct cataracts, glaucoma and the like. On the surface, it sounds crazy, but it made more and more sense once I dove into what we know of the science of hair, what works, what doesn't and why. Surprisingly, there is a significant amount of overlap between the devices and medications used for hair growth already in use in an average ophthalmologist's office, on the effects of hormones on the end target and the results of unchecked inflammation on hair growth and on eye health. Some of it was new like Rogaine and finasteride but many of the cornerstone hair growth medications are already being used by eye doctors. Latisse, light therapy, lasers and the principles of microsurgery are squarely in the wheelhouse of ophthalmologists, so I had more familiarity than I even imagined with most of therapies before I even got started in the hair business.

I personally became involved in hair restoration through my work with the NFL cheerleaders in my area. They are contractually obligated to wear beautiful (and expensive) hair and lash extensions so they look extra gorgeous on the field and off. They wear their extensions 24/7 through the season with all the normal wear and tear plus they perform all kinds of sexy hair flips during their halftime routines that pull and create traction. Both their hair and lash extensions ultimately took their toll on the natural hair. At the end of the season, a lot of them had hair that was broken, weakened, even pulled out by the root. And they weren't the only ones participating in the lash extension craze – it had gone mainstream by that point. What I noticed was no matter how skilled your lash artist, eventually those beautiful lash extensions will take their toll. The artificial lashes add weight onto natural lashes causing weakening and breakage (sometimes down to the base of lash!) and the glue used to affix them causes eye irritation and chemical damage resulting in thin, brittle eyelashes. I had already been treating dry eye related to lash extensions, ocular allergies and reactions to glue, corneal abrasions when the lashes fell into the eye and eye irritation related to extensions and now I found myself doing eyelash rehab in their off-season, primarily with Latisse and products like it. Of course, they wanted to know if what was helping their eyelashes would also help the hair on their head. (Spoiler alert: it does.)

Next, I myself experienced a more stressful than normal year. In fairness, some of it could have been hormonal, too. I started noticing that my hair was clogging the drain in the bathtub. At any given time, I could dredge up enough hair on my bathroom floor after blow drying to create my own tiny American Girl doll wig. It was time to do what I do best: dive into the research, rely on scientific studies and start separating the marketing and hype from the science. I used this process to create a family of proven scientific solutions to solve this problem for my patients, for myself and anyone else who suffers from unwanted hair loss or thinning and wanted to learn more about preventing it.

The truth is, almost everyone has or will run into a hair los at some point. The numbers tell the story: by the age of 35, 66% of American men will experience some degree of noticeable hair loss.[1] 35! That's still pretty young to resign yourself to letting go. The numbers for women are maybe more disturbing because it's not culturally acceptable to just shave your head and get on with your life. Twenty one million women currently suffer with alopecia and 80% of women will have noticeable hair loss in their lifetimes.[2] Hair loss in both men and women can start as early as the 20s and even the teenage years and the psychological and social implications can be severe.

A little about me. You should know that I am impatient by nature and appreciate the instant and miraculous results of LASIK, cataract surgery and some of the non-invasive facial rejuvenation techniques that I have grown to love like MIXTOLaserLift. I am not typically satisfied with results that I have to squint at to appreciate. There are some things in life that cannot be modified but with everything I've learned I do not believe that genetics and the progression of time does not have to dictate your hairline. I am ready to share what I've learned here so that we can use science together to achieve the hair that you always wanted or the hair you never had.

Here at Toyos Clinic we have almost every type of solution that exists for unwanted hair loss that I will describe to you now. Pick what you like: some people prefer only non-invasive solutions, others like to do everything possible – all at the same time, and there are some others that go straight to surgery knowing that they will never keep up with vitamins or topicals on a day to basis. My job is to show you what's out there that can help, help you understand how much it can help and it will be your job to choose the product or products that feel right for you. The following list of solutions that I will describe to you is the closest I have found to LASIK for hair – and the results are definitely worth it.

Jessi's story

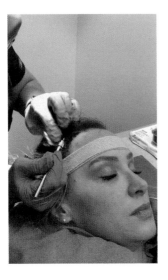

I'm a professional dancer, actress, and model. You may have seen me dancing for some of the biggest names in pop and country music or the . Basically, I make my living on the stage and screen. Ive been in the public eye since I was a teenager. At about 19 years old I first noticed the recession of the two sides of my hairline. It started off slowly but kept going until I had two deep "v"s on the side of my face. I stopped wearing my hair back in a ponytail which had also begun to thin and started getting creative with the way I styled my hair. I definitely went through a phase of "why me?" Like many women who suffer from hair loss, it was hard to maintain my confidence. Being in front of the camera exacerbated my insecurities and I knew I had to do something.

I spent hours in front of the mirror, scrutinizing my scalp from this way and that, trying to camouflage everything, praying and wondering how bad it would ultimately get. I got paranoid thinking everyone I spoke to was staring at my forehead and noticed the thinning hair. Sometimes I cancelled plans with friends because I just didn't feel up to it.

Even though I knew better, part of me hoped it was all in my head and no one noticed the way I did. My bubble burst one day while getting my hair done. My hairdresser started questioning me about overusing my straightener and curling iron, wearing my ponytail too tight, and buying cheap styling products. She assumed these practices were causing my hair to thin and fall out. I went home and cried. Shortly after, I decided to get the triangular shaped bald areas of my hairline tattooed with color. It's called scalp micropigmentation. I knew a few European soccer stars who'd had it done. Unfortunately it has to be touched up multiple times a year and it's as painful as any confluent tattoo would be. It took a couple of days to recover from the pain of the procedure. The final result was less than favorable. Yes, there was color on my scalp (just like hair) and I didn't have to worry about covering it up all the time. But it looked more like a brownish red shadow that was cast on my skin, not actual hair. It helped a bit but, it wasn't a permanent solution.

Still unsatisfied, I searched for options. Hormone replacement wasn't appealing as a young woman (under 30) and not willing to risk negatively affecting my ability to have children.

 Finally, I found SmartGraft! It seemed like the perfect solution for me! I have long hair so the donor site that had to be shaved was completely covered. It takes time for the shorter hair in that area to grow and catch up to the rest but, it's not noticeable at all. Even when dancing with a ponytail! The grafts were done (just 500) last November over the top of my tattooed skin and now that area looks even better. My hairdresser recently commented how much nicer my hairline looks. After the procedure there were a few days of treating the grafts gently, but I was able to work from home and didn't need any help after surgery. I would do it again if I needed to and I would absolutely recommend it for anyone who is feeling self-conscious about their hair the way I was.

Hair Loss: The Causes

The statistics tell us that most people will face unwelcome changes in their hair at some point in their lives. It might be massive shedding after pregnancy, a slow realization of hair thinning or loss, or even a gradual loss of the shininess and luster you took for granted in your youth. With age, hair follicles naturally become smaller resulting in less coverage even if you aren't losing hair and the hair that does grow begins to grow at a slower rate and with less natural gloss. As we begin your hair recovery journey, it's important that you start by seeing your medical doctor to rule out medical causes of hair problems that can affect your overall health.

It's normal to lose between 50-100 hairs per day. Most doctors will start by having you collect hair from your brush or the floor and they or you can literally count it to see where you fall on the spectrum. Sometimes longer hair falling out can actually look like more hair because there is more of it. What I have typically found is that if you feel are noticing more hair than normal in the drain after washing your hair, more on the floor after blow drying or are removing larger amounts than normal in your brush, you probably do have a hair situation on your hands.   It is a fact that you can lose up to 50% of your hair density before it becomes noticeable. Soooo, by the time you notice that you have a problem, more than likely your suspicions are correct. By far and away, the most common cause of hair loss is hereditary male and female pattern hair loss related to age (birthdays, I always say). It is true that hair loss is typically dictated by the males on the maternal side of the family, but if hair loss runs in your family generally, you are more likely to experience it too. Like Andre Agassi, hair loss can start as early as puberty – I see plenty of college aged patients in my office often along with their parents eager to avoid or at least delay the fates of their relatives.

Both female and male pattern baldness runs in families but they lose their hair in different ways. Men tend to lose hair from the temples (frontal recession) and from the crown of the head. Women usually notice a more diffuse loss across the top of the head and often notice a widening of the part or "flattening" at the top. They can notice recession of the entire hairline or just the sides as well.

Hormones and any changes related to them can cause abrupt changes in hair. Pregnancy, childbirth, polycystic ovary disease, and even discontinuing birth control pills can all cause an impromptu and horrifying shedding of hair as the hairs that were primed to linger in the growth phase during the hormonal influence suddenly return to their more normal, staggered growth cycles. Crash dieting can also lead to hair loss.

Anytime you cut way back on your calories or nutrition – especially protein, your body will eliminate "non-essential services" including hair maintenance and growth. In most of these cases, it takes about 90 days of normalization of calories and eating patterns for the body to pick back up where it left off.

There are plenty of common medications that are known for contributing to hair loss. The list includes blood thinners such as warfarin, Accutane which is commonly used for acne, amphetamines, antidepressants specifically Prozac and Zoloft (which are found in our water supply in small but measurable quantities), beta blockers used for high blood pressure and anxiety and cholesterol lowering drugs like Lipitor. Lithium and Parkinson's medications are all known to contribute to hair loss. Chemotherapy for cancer is obviously a cause of hair loss. Your doctor can help you determine if substitutions can be made or dosages adjusted. Hair loss due to medication typically begins to reverse once the offending medication is discontinued.

And let us not overlook stress. Stress is a common cause of hair shedding, too. This condition has a name: telogen effluvium. Severe emotional distress, fever, illness and marked weight loss can all contribute to noticeable hair loss as the body makes an executive decision to eliminate processes like hair growth that it feels are extraneous to survival. This type of hair loss can occur over several weeks to months but recovers over the following 3-6 months once the stress of the situation has lifted. Of course, losing hair by itself causes stress, so there is always the possibility of getting caught up in that downward spiral.

Your medical doctor will sure that your hair loss isn't related to a medical disorder like thyroid dysfunction, fungal infection, autoimmune reaction, hormone imbalances, polycystic ovary disease or a dietary deficiency. One autoimmune disease, alopecia areata, which commonly affects young women is particularly distressing and causes areas of hair including eyebrows and eyelashes to fall out suddenly. These areas of patchy hair loss can appear on the scalp to be similar to "crop circles" circular or semicircular areas with sharp edges of complete hair loss. Because this is a disease that is caused by the body attacking its own hair follicles, it can be treated with steroids, steroid injections and other immunomodulators.

What else causes hair loss? Certain hair products and styles. One big cause are hair extensions. Ironic, because most people seek extensions because they want thick, full hair. Extensions by definition cause traction, pull and break hair further worsening the hair loss. The cycle can be vicious, with people seeking even more extensions as they worsen the underlying issue. Traction related damage can also be caused by certain hairstyles including too tight ponytails. Tight braids, buns, ponytails, and cornrows can all cause the hair to break right at the scalp, causing breakage which can take years to recover.

Too much processing: excessive heat, bleaching, tugging on your hair when it's wet and vulnerable and multiple processes can weaken natural hair, as well. One word of caution: never apply heat to wet hair and use the lowest heat settings possible to protect your precious hair. If you happen to notice steam coming off your hair, it's waaayy too hot. Try to stay away from the 300-400 degree range on your flatiron if at all possible. Remember that the hair you see is already dead and cannot repair itself once damaged (one caveat: Olaplex products which we will cover in a later section). This type of damage generally has to be cut off in order to prevent the breakage and splitting from moving further upstream. Once more normal styling practices are instituted, traction or damage alopecia will begin to subside.

Hair Loss Treatment: A Brief and Amusing History

Most people that suffer from hair loss feel pretty alone in their misery even with the statistics that tell us otherwise. The truth is that people have been trying to fix their hair problems since back in the times of the ancient peoples. Because they didn't yet have the understanding of the causes and roots of hair loss, the solutions that they dreamed up probably seem a little strange to the modern reader. But honestly, if someone told you they absolutely had the answer to hair loss, is there anything you wouldn't try?

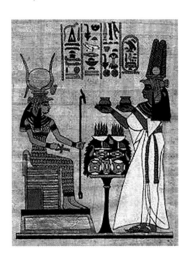

First, the Egyptians. There are many hieroglyphics that have been preserved that show hair care and treatments, signifying its importance during those times. They are also responsible for writing the oldest and first known prescription for baldness is known as the Ebers Papyrus, written in 1550 BC. This paper scroll and early medical writing offered a number of possible solutions for early Egyptian men and women suffering from hair loss. The recipes called for mixing an iron oxide found in the ground with lead, onions, honey and alabaster then slowly folding in fat from a variety of animals. The sufferer could take their choice from hippopotamuses, crocodiles, ibexes, tomcats, or snakes. This literal snake oil cure (no relation to the salesmen that came later) for hair loss was to designed to be ingested orally but only after the patient appealed to the Sun God Ra calling out "Oh, shining one, who hoverest above!"[3] They had other far-fetched ideas, too, like boiling porcupine hair in water and applying daily to affected areas for four days and sauteeing the leg of a greyhound together with a donkey hoof. There's no record of how often these treatments achieved their desired outcomes but the early Egyptians were known to be early and frequent users of wigs and fake beards.[4]

The next great thinker of the ages in the world of hair loss was none other than Hippocrates, the Father of Western Medicine himself, an original OG Greek physician. Born in 460 BC, Hippocrates was a famous teacher and physician known in his time as he is now for his enduring ethical and philosophical approach to medicine. He connected annual records of weather with associated diseases in his work Epidemics, explained how to set fractures and treat wounds and even delved into preventative care. Despite all of these successes, he was known to be short in stature and personally struggled with hair loss. For this, he prescribed for himself and others topical mixtures of opium (which likely only lessened the psychological pain of baldness), horseradish, pigeon droppings, beets and assorted spices. He also correctly observed that members of the Persian Army guarding the King's harem did not experience hair loss if they had been castrated before the age of 25. In 1995, hair researchers at Duke University confirmed that castration in fact does prevent baldness but I suspect this method is not likely to catch on given the current availability of treatments.[5]

Next up in history was Julius Caesar himself, the famous Roman dictator and lover of Cleopatra lived from 100 BC to 44 BC. In the ultimate mullet gone wrong, by necessity he ended up growing his hair long in the back and combing it over the top (insert Donald Trump joke). Cleopatra tried and failed to help him by suggesting her own concoction of ground up mice, horse teeth, and bear grease. Ultimately, Caesar began to wear the laurel wreath, symbol of success, full time and not just on special occasions. Presumably the switch occurred to symbolize his status as a strong and powerful leader but one can't help but notice, it also conveniently covered up his bald spots.[6]

For reasons probably related to the idea of fertilizer or maybe just the thought that the grosser the treatment, the more likely it was to work, a variety of excretions or poop, if you will, were tried by those seeking hair restoration. A physician in ancient Rome recommended that patients treat their hair loss by burning the genitals of a donkey, mixing the genital ash with the patient's own urine and applying the paste topically the needed areas. No less than Aristotle himself, the great Greek philosopher, purportedly regularly applied goat urine to his scalp and perfected the art of the forward combover for his sculptures.

In terms of urine, there might be a scientific rationale behind the madness of using urine as a hair loss treatment. Urine from males of all species is known to contain measurable levels of testosterone. Perhaps that is why King Henry the Eighth was said to prefer dog and horse urine, and Native American Indians applied chicken and cow manure topically. Other times, there was less scientific explanation to be had and it seemed that people simply used what they had available at the time. Like in the 19th century, when the British took to applying "cold India tea" and lemons to their balding heads. In America, the shysters and "snake oil" salesmen were out in full force in the 19th century, but their products of choice were hot peppers and Spanish fly, meant to improve circulation and virility. The early 20th century ventured more into an industrial phase and saw mechanical devices being manufactured as treatments like the blue-light, heat-emitting Thermocap (an early precursor for to hair cap for growth like Capillus?). Men and women were instructed to spend 15 minutes daily under the cap for optimal growth. Glowing electrically powered glass combs were tried with limited success and finally a vacuum was invented in order to use suction to coax dormant hair follicles out of the scalp. The vacuum systems could be widely found in barbershops or rented for more discreet at home use. Natural herbal and ayurvedic treatments were also being tried, some of which are still in use today. Products like cold-pressed castor oil which has a small amount of prostaglandin activity, almond oil, coconut milk, fenugreek seeds, licorice root, beets (Hippocrates was right!), onion (Caesar was too!), aloe vera and a compound made from the gooseberry called Amla that is this very day being used by the newest Bumble and Bumble hair care thickening line.[7]

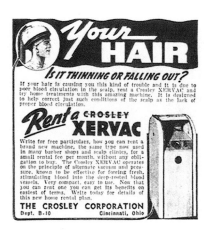

It was the Japanese that came up the foundations of modern hair transplant surgery and thanks to the World War that was going on, the world almost never learned about it. In 1939, Dr. Shoji Okuda successfully pioneered a procedure transferring hair from the back of the scalp onto patient's bald spots. Unlike Caucasian men, Asian men have historically experienced the lowest rates of hair loss in the world. Less than 15% of all men ever develop any hair loss (remember it was 66% of US men) and when they do develop baldness, it occurs roughly a decade later than other Western societies. With such low rates, this has developed into something of a cultural stigma with the added impetus for physicians to find a cure. It is no wonder that this technique first arose in the Asian world. The discovery remained hidden from the scientific community for over two decades until the documentation of these procedures were found and shared and a New York doctor, by the name of Norman Orentreich, at the insistence of a particularly persuasive male pattern baldness patient, began to perform and popularize the punch graft procedure.[8] And the rest, as they say, is history.

Vitamins and Supplements: What Works, What Doesn't from A to Zinc

There are so many products on the shelves that claim to promote hair growth. Some are just common sense. Some are things that have been repeated so often they are believed to be true (i.e. biotin) and a many are just hype. Here we are going to talk about diet, supplements and what science says are the best products to fill in the gaps in your diet and wellness so that you can make your own hair grow thicker and fuller and even improve the texture of your hair with the foods you choose.

Let's talk about your diet. With our busy lives and specific dietary requirements (vegan, vegetarian, flexitarian) it can be hard to get everything we need for health in general on a daily basis let alone for optimal hair growth. Hair is one of the fastest growing and dividing cells in our body and any consequently, any nutritional shortcomings will often show up here first. Most of the vitamin and supplement recommendations center around a few key ideas: promoting the collagen building process, reducing inflammation and improving circulation-- especially microcirculation around hair follicles needed to deliver oxygen and key building blocks like amino acids.

The rate our hair grows can be genetically determined (some people's hair just grows faster than others) but generally hair growth slows down as we age – that's part of why it becomes harder to maintain longer hairstyles. Theoretically hair should grow about a half inch per month - 6 inches total in a year[9] and ingesting the right micronutrients can be key to the success of healthy growing hair. Five trace elements have been found to be critical for healthy hair. The first is biotin, one of the B vitamins – with a few caveats. Biotin supplements can be found on any grocery store shelf promoting hair and nail growth. Biotin supplements have literally been ingrained in our minds as critical for these functions – the advertising has worked and everybody knows to look for biotin - but in truth, for healthy adults, the data is that supplementation would help an already healthy person is scarce. Biotin deficiency clearly causes hair loss but that is uncommon in our world except in cases of alcoholism and severe malnutrition but sometimes, people can be subtly deficient and not realize it. The recommended daily allowance of biotin calls for most adults to consume about 20 mcg – easily found in one egg, a cup of milk, or a handful of almonds. Some vitamins like vitamin A can cause toxicity when taken to excess. I've never seen a biotin overdose per se and I am unaware of any serious detrimental effect that could occur with overdosing. Biotin seems to be processed in the system within about 8 hours with half of any excess being excreted in the urine and half in the stool. Bottom line: taking extra biotin may help your hair and taking a little extra probably won't hurt you. Don't count on dramatic results but every little bit can help. Next up is zinc – which is shown to grow and repair hair naturally. Zinc has made a name for itself warding off colds and other viruses like COVID-19, but it's also an important cofactor in hair growth. True zinc deficiency is known to lead to hair loss but zinc also contributes hair health by supporting the oil glands around the hair that keep hair supple. Just like biotin, true zinc deficiency is rare but relative deficiency may be more prevalent when people restrict their diets, reducing or eliminating red meat, dairy. Pregnancy is an independent risk factor as well. Dietary zinc is found in meat, dairy, whole grains and nuts. The third micronutrient is copper which curbs some of the hormones that can lead to hair loss as well as being a critical co-factor in microcirculation, hair growth and boosting collagen and elastin production in skin. Iron is number four and also one of the most common deficiencies I see in women due to menstruation, childbearing and restriction of red meat ingestion. Blood tests will show it but in the office, I generally pull their lower lip and/or lower eyelid out to look to see if their mucous membranes are getting a little pale. If so, I absolutely recommend prenatal vitamins (most regular vitamins don't have iron or enough iron) and/or an iron supplement. The iron gluconate supplement is the easiest one to ingest with less stomach irritation and GI side effects than the iron sulfates. I usually ask patients if they've been feeling a little run down and/or short of breath with exercise which are also common symptoms. Getting the right amount of iron is important for another reason in hair growth: iron makes up the hemoglobin in red blood cells that helps to get oxygen and nutrition to growing hair. Eat your spinach or if you aren't a fan of green leafy vegetables, at least take your supplement for healthy hair growth. I learned during my own pregnancies that Cream of Wheat has a surprising amount of iron in it and is a little more appealing sometimes than a bowl of spinach. Lastly, selenium is an often overlooked micronutrient needed for optimal hair growing. Selenium is found in meat, nuts, cereals and mushrooms and helps to reduce inflammation and oxidative damage done by stress and pollution. There is some evidence that selenium supplementation can even inhibit certain autoimmune diseases including Hashimoto's, a thyroid condition.[10]

Protein. Some of my cosmetic patients are bodybuilders who make it their business to eat large amounts of animal protein daily to build their muscles. You can't help but notice that many of them also have thick, lush hair. When I ask about their diets, they are eating lots of animal sourced protein, drinking branched chain amino acids (the building blocks of protein), and basically feeding their bodies hair food all day long. This is the reason for their strong hair game. Hair is made of protein so all of the amino acids are important. There are, however, a few amino acids (the building blocks of protein) that are particularly essential for strong, healthy hair. Cysteine and methionine are perfect examples - both of them are absolutely necessary for hair growth. Cysteine grows hair and stimulates new hair growth, the sulfur in it helps to build critical disulfide bridges that are responsible for your hair's shape and strength (we will talk later about Olaplex, another hair care line, that contains a disulfide bridge multiplier to help repair damaged hair) to not only build hair, but to also repair damaged hair and improve the texture and tensile strength of the hair. As if that weren't enough, natural supplementation of cysteine acts as a strong anti-oxidant to help protect against environmental assaults and sun damage. Supplementation with oral cysteine has been shown to be helpful even in patients with alopecia. The next sulfur containing amino acid, methionine, you're going to love for a couple of reasons: it grows hair, improves microcirculation to the hair and scalp, strengthens hair and *helps prevent fat accumulation in specific body areas.* More hair and less fat? No wonder the bodybuilders love it. Yes, please.[11]

Collagen deserves a special discussion all on its own. Recently, powdered collagen has become popular as an additive to improve skin and hair. Specifically, marine sourced peptides dumped into smoothies or cups of yogurt has been touted as a cure all for hair, skin, nails, bone, and joint health. A pretty tall order with little to no science to back it up. There is some data that shows improvement in both the bones and the hair of mice when given orally as well as enhanced wound healing.[12] Initially, I was a skeptic. You know what else is made of collagen? Fried pork rinds made from the skin of pigs – which were cheaper and looked to me like they would be similarly effective. Then I learned than in Japan, that young women were buying dried animal skins to chew on them to gain the cosmetic benefits of ingested collagen.[13] Much like the chew toys that you might purchase for your pets, except more expensive and for people. So is it worth it or no? Although the collagen craze is something of a fad, it does provide a source of amino acids that many people need. I would have to say worth it for sure if you aren't getting enough protein in your regular diet. Many women are not. Thanks to my body building friends, I do believe that having extra "bonus" amino acids in your system not needed for muscle repair, et cetera are going to be available for use in growing hair. So, since I'm not a fan of pork rinds, or chew toys if I'm honest, I personally consume two scoops of marine sourced collagen daily. Another reasonable alternative for my non-vegan friends is to drink your collagen by consuming bone broth. Bone broth is made by simmering animal bones (usually chicken, turkey or beef) for 8-24 hours to extract the maximum amount of flavor and nutritional benefits. Bone broth can be enjoyed either alone or used in soups or in the cooking of whole grains like quinoa. Because the materials are already partially broken down and ready to easily digest, it is a readily bioavailable source chock full of collagen, protein, amino acids and minerals.

Antioxidants go hand in hand with protein because your body needs vitamin C to carry out collagen production (a big part of hair growing) as well as to protect hair, scalp and follicles from environmental or other stressors that can create oxidizing particles that damage hair or scalp and prevent against premature aging or damage. Antioxidants help you build and maintain strong healthy hair. All anti-oxidants: vitamin C, vitamin E and green tea extracts (the mother of all anti-oxidants) specifically help prevent the production of and limit the damage of any existing free radicals. Free radicals are unstable molecules that cause damage to cells when triggered by stress, pollution and well, just life.

Other lesser known supplements can also be helpful as well. Ingredients like horsetail rush, MSM, and gamma linolenic acid are strongly anti-inflammatory to combat the toxins of everyday life that take a toll on your skin and hair. Grapeseed extract is naturally anti-bacterial in case your normal balance has been disrupted. Saw palmetto and other plant-based ingredients that can offset hormonal imbalances that can cause hair loss and thinning.

Another specific vitamin supplement tied to hair loss and hair regrowth is Vitamin D. Vitamin D is known to be connected to hair growth, the creation of new hair follicles and maintenance of the thickness of individual hair strands. Vitamin D and zinc deficiencies have also been loosely connected with alopecia areata. You're likely not getting enough vitamin D sitting inside at your office job, so adding a supplement is good for your health and your hair. [14]

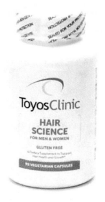

Lastly, the cells of hair bulb follicle divide every 23 to 72 hours, significantly faster than any other cell on the body. Because of that, it is imperative that patients seeking the best hair regrowth results receive enough vitamin A and B complex vitamins to support this rapid growth. Food sources of vitamin A are carrots (of course), cantaloupe, spinach and sweet potatoes. B vitamins specifically help carry oxygen and nutrients to the scalp and hair follicles.[15] B vitamins are found in salmon, leafy greens and eggs.

A special word about vitamin B12. Because of a study showing beneficial effects in pain reduction in patients with dry eye, our clinic recently began to offer vitamin B12 shots to those patients. I have a daughter who is vegan and very likely does not get enough B12 in her diet but I was surprised to learn that other very commonly used medications interfere with the absorption of B12 in the diet like birth control pills, over the counter stomach acid medications like Prilosec, metformin (a drug commonly used in diabetes), consumption of alcohol and allergy medications. Is there anyone who doesn't think they might be deficient now? On top of all that, we slowly lose the ability to absorb B12 in our food so that by the time we are 70, our natural absorption is almost zero. I began to offer B12 shots to my hair patients as well as my dry eye patients. B12 is critical in bringing needed nutrients to the active hair follicle and just like protein, I believe in providing all of the building blocks needed for hair growth and maybe just a little extra to make sure there is enough to go around and plenty extra left over for hair growing[16].

I always believe that consuming our nutrients in food is preferable to supplementation but it's tough to get everything we need every single day. Growing hair takes consistency so I created our medical-grade, bio-optimized hair supplement HairScience for use every day based on the scientific studies I reviewed using ingredients proven to grow hair. We even made our formulation vegan and gluten free for those with dietary restrictions. A few improvements and adjustments to your diet, plus a dietary hair supplement and a good prenatal are all easy to incorporate. Diet and nutritional supplements are one of most accessible methods for starting to grow the hair of your dreams. More hair and better hair awaits!

Cost for supplements: 10-200 dollars/month.

Linda's story

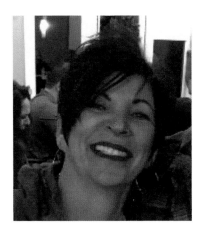 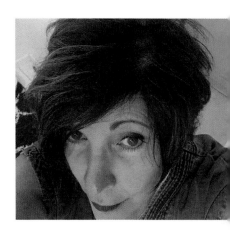

My hair fell out when I hit menopause.

You have to understand that I'm Lebanese and have always had thick, lustrous hair. So thick that in my 20's I could barely get a brush through all of it, it runs in my family. So you can't even imagine my surprise when I started noticing dark hair on the carpet (mine) and the mat of hair that clogged my bathroom drain after I washed it. I started comparing the amount of hair in my hairbrush with the previous day. It got better then worse as I worked with my doctor to start taking hormonal treatments for menopause. One combination of hormones caused so much shedding, I started seeing my hairline recede and my part widening by the day. To most people, I have a lot of hair – still. But to me, knowing what was typical for me this was a massive shock. I had no way of knowing how far it would go or how bad it would get. Would I end of with bald patches?

I started wearing my hair different ways, parting it over the thinning part, brushing it forward. It was depressing! I know I'm getting older, but I don't feel old and don't think I look my age. I wanted to keep that going. I tried a couple of shampoos made for thinning hair and really didn't notice a difference. I bought a light cap which totally helps. It's easy to wear around the house and I work from home anyway but I still wanted more which is how I ended up talking to Dr. Toyos about other options. I was interested in the hair transplant surgery but after she examined me, she decided I didn't need it. I started taking the HairScience vitamins and noticed a difference right away – my hair and my nails, they were growing so fast I had to cut them every two weeks just to keep up. My hair started looking really nice, too. At first, I thought the improvements might be all in my head but then I started getting compliments. Other people were noticing it, too.

She also gave me some of the Rogaine Plus too. I use that once or twice a day and after the first month I noticed lots of new little hairs growing especially around the hairline. I'm thrilled. I've gotten my hormones on a more even keel now and that seems to have helped as well.

I know that I'm not alone. I've spoken to a lot of women my age who have some version of this same story. But I didn't want to just let it get worse. My hair is part of who I am. It's always been something that I was proud of – that people noticed about me. I'm really glad that I've found a combination of treatments that works for me and I'm going to stick with it so my hair will stick with me!

Topicals: Rogaine and Beyond

Prescription topical products for hair loss remain something of a mystery. Many of them are standard of care and have literally been used for decades to grow hair without ever really understanding the mechanisms by which these medicines actually work.

For example, the most commonly recognized topical medication is Rogaine, an old blood pressure medicine. It has been generically produced for years since its approval in 1996. It comes in two strengths: 2% and 5%. You can even now find it on store shelves like Costco. Long felt to be just for men, now even the stronger 5% concentration is routinely used for women's hair loss and has been proven to be more effective than the 2% dose. Please note that the generically produced label states that it is only for men as that was the case when Rogaine was approved. Label changes are multi-million dollars ventures and companies are not likely to recoup their costs with a generic medication. Therefore, the label has, is and will always states "For Men Only" even though it has become standard practice in the treatment of female pattern hair loss.

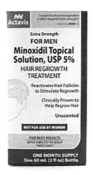

Women can use Rogaine at any point in their lives, not just postmenopausal hair loss but women who are considering pregnancy should avoid minoxidil during pregnancy and breastfeeding because of the risk of birth defects. [17] The benefit of Rogaine is not just in its ability to grow hair when applied topically but to increase the diameter of the hair follicle itself. This serves two purposes: one to reverse the miniaturization that occurs with age and to improve the coverage of the scalp with the existing hair. It also extends the hair growth cycle allowing hair to grow for a longer period of time, resulting in more hair growth. (This growth boost is particularly helpful if you feel your hair growth "hits a wall," slows down or just doesn't seem to want to grow past a certain length.)

No one knows all of the mechanisms triggered by Rogaine to grow hair, but this much is clear: it increases the amount of blood circulating in the scalp around the hair follicle, it lengthens the growth phase of the hair which helps you grow longer, thicker hair and it widens the hair follicle itself. It remains the only over the counter hair growth product the FDA has approved for head hair growth and the only topical product approved by the FDA. It works pretty quickly: studies show about 25% more hair within 90 days. It works for most people, too – 9 out 10 men noticed improvement when used twice daily for four months. It has been approved for male and female pattern hair loss and is commonly used for eyebrow and beard enhancement as well as other hair deficiency issues. The available studies show that Rogaine has been proven effective for hair loss in the front and the back for women but only in the back for men.[18] Having said that, you should know that the original study for Rogaine only focused on the crown area of the scalp and did not address the improvements on the hairline. Most hair specialists have seen Rogaine work on the hairlines of men, so please know that it works but because this medicine is now generic, it is is unlikely that further studies or label changes will occur. This is the same reason that some generic Rogaine label will say "Not for women" – that was the knowledge at the time of approval, and no one is anxious to spend millions of dollars on a label change when it is already being used for both men and women in practice.

When combined with topical vitamin A, Rogaine becomes even more powerful, increasing its potency by 153% according to one study. Used together, the two medications both extend the hair growth signaling pathway and downregulate pathways associated with hair and scalp cell death.[19] Win-win-win. We have always utilized a nanomicellular vitamin A or retinol in order to enhance absorption and penetration for skin care and co-opted our very own IScience retinol for use with Rogaine that we mix together in the office. Nanomicelles are tiny, self-assembling particles in which medication is generally embedded within the center of the sphere. Smaller medication particles increase surface area in order to allow better and faster absorption, potency and penetration of medication to the target tissues. Vitamin A, long a staple of skin care, is known to be a useful adjunct for scalp care and hair growth because all cells need vitamin A for growth, especially the fast growing hair follicles.. Adding topical vitamin A **alone** can increase hair growth by 60%.[20] Vitamin A itself is known to be drying to the skin and scalp but the nanomicellular version only requires a tiny amount to be useful and is quickly soaked into the scalp so we see few side effects from this formulation. Vitamin A also boosts cell turnover, reverses some of the processes of aging and promotes new cell growth. Adding Vitamin A to the Rogaine solution increases the potency so much that the normal formula can be used once daily instead of twice. However, when patients want the fastest results possible, I tell my patients that "once daily works and twice daily works faster."[21]

Prostaglandins like Latisse are another integral part of topical hair growth products. Originally marketed as glaucoma eye drops, I remember my surprise and astonishment 20 years ago when senior citizens returned to our eye clinics for their glaucoma eye pressure checks with long, thick glossy eyelashes. Their lashes were so long, they often got in the way of surgery and patients were begging us in the clinics to cut their eyelashes because they had grown so long they were rubbing against their glasses. It was a "problem" that turned out to have a pretty significant market value when the same company patented the right to sell the same medication as Latisse, the lash growing topically applied medication but for whatever reason, it never got past Phase I clinical trials for the the treatment of alopecia.

At any given time, an average person has about 100,000 hairs on their heads with approximately 90% in the active growth phase called anagen. Hair normally grows in a 3-4 month cycle: growth, resting, falling out, and getting ready to grow again. Prostaglandins are like the Jillian Michaels of hair care because they have the ability to coax all available hair follicles off the couch and into the active growth mode, effectively doubling the density of the hair within a few weeks' time. Prostaglandins also cause hypertrophic (literally big growth) changes: hairs grow longer, thicker and darker. Prostaglandins are the same hormone that causes women to experience dense, thick hair during pregnancy. However, unlike pregnancy, these products can be used and maintained continuously in order to keep hair follicles in the growth mode.[22] The main thing to remember is that only a tiny bit is needed and these products grow hair wherever they are used -so use them judiciously! There are many products in this family that go by many names; bimatoprost, travaprost, latanoprost, the list goes on.[23] Latisse is reported to work in about 70% of patients using it and it is believed that an active hair follicle must be present for it to stimulate in order to work i.e. scarred or dead follicles cannot be brought back to life. There are potential side effects that mirror the side effects when these products are used for lash growth namely: skin discoloration (actually could be positive if you have darker hair) and minor local irritation.

There are a few other products that are known to grow hair. One category is immune modulators believed to downregulate a body's overactive immune response that leads to a body attacking its own hair follicles. There is significant evidence to show that inflammation plays an important role in hair loss. We've known for a long time that autoimmune diseases (that primarily affect women) are associated with hair loss. Because of my work with dry eye, I know that many more are affected with subclinical inflammation that has not or not yet been diagnosed but can absolutely produce noticeable symptoms. Now there in new research to suggest that specific autoimmune cells are connected to hair follicles that are dead or dying. Reining in the inflammation with anti-inflammatories and immunomodulators is absolutely a wide-open new pathway to reversing hair loss.

Our original experiences with anti-inflammatories were in people with known autoimmune diseases like alopecia areata. Topical and injected steroids have been known to improve hair growth in the autoimmune condition alopecia areata. Steroids are not practical for long term use because they have any number of side effects from scalp thinning, irritation, insomnia, bruising and susceptibility to certain infections.[24]

One immunomodulatory currently in use that holds significant promise is cyclosporine. Cyclosporine is more commonly known in the marketplace as Restasis, used to treat dry eye for over a decade and known to grow hair since the 1960s. Cyclosporine is officially a calcineurin inhibitor, an immunosuppressant and modulator and may help to grow hair by reducing the body's propensity to attack its own hair follicles. For a topical medication in use for hair loss since the 60s, the research is fairly light. So far, we only know that it inhibits a hair suppressor, slows down programmed hair cell death, reduces autoimmune activity directed at hair follicles and increases a number of growth factors that influence hair growth.[25] It also increases the number of available hair follicles and extends the hair growth cycle.[26] Although it has some of the same results, cyclosporine works in a completely different way than Rogaine and in fact, can grow hair in situations where Rogaine cannot, even in some cases alopecia areata.[27] Luckily for us, cyclosporine has now also been produced as a nanomicellular molecule (Cequa, Sun Pharmaceuticals) to enhance the tissue penetration into the scalp and effectivity of the molecule at the target site.[28]

Anti-fungal products have also long been known to be useful in hair growth. Most people are familiar with these products as the feminine anti-yeast vaginal creams found on the store shelves of drug stores and grocery stores. Pharmacies and veterinary outlets are able to produce or create anti-fungal solutions that are more conducive to topical hair products than a thick, white ointment and may work by reducing the overgrowth of normal fungi appearing on scalps and skin surfaces. It doesn't work as well as Rogaine itself, but it can be a helpful addition to the mix to help boost the effect of Rogaine alone.[29]

What else? There is a little bit of evidence that lavender oil, sandolore (derivative of sandalwood) and maybe even peppermint oil may help with hair follicle development, depth of hair follicle development and scalp thickness (thicker scalps are better anchors and provide more nutrition for growing hair). Lavender oil also showed that it reduced certain types of inflammatory cells that might, if misdirected, attack hair follicles to the detriment of hair growing. It certainly can help a hair formula smell nice and fresh, but a not much is needed as a little bit goes a long way.

We created our formula called Rogaine Plus to take advantage of all of the topicals that have been proven to grow hair. Starting with a base of 5% Rogaine, I mix (under a fume hood) in prostaglandin, cyclosporine and retinol to pump up the effectivity of the already effective Rogaine with a dash of lavendar. I haven't yet done any controlled clinical trials but anecdotally patients report noticeable hair growth starting between 30- 90 days. One package contains two 60 ml bottles or two to four months' supply or more depending on how you use it. I recommend using 1 ml once or twice daily to moisten the areas that need growth. I personally prefer the liquid minoxidil to the foam as the foam causes a "crunchy" effect at the roots of hair that is annoying to me. I also like that the formulation is small enough to stash in my purse and that I don't have to worry about traveling with it.

Cost: 32 for generic Rogaine or 250 for 3-4 months of Rogaine Plus

Emitt's Story

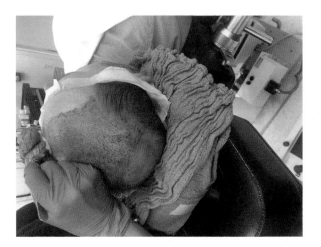

Every man in my family has hair loss so growing up, it wasn't really a question of if for me, but when. Turns out, I had just turned 20 when I first saw the signs. I'm not really one for complicated beauty routines, basically I jump in the shower with some soap and shampoo and I'm out the door. I normally wouldn't even take time to brush my hair, just run my fingers through it before heading out and that's when I first started noticing more dark hairs in my hands than I was used to seeing. At first, I thought that I was having a reaction to my girlfriend's fancy shampoo so I grabbed the cheaper brand that I normally used next time I was as the grocery store but that didn't seem to help.

I went on like that for a while until one day my girlfriend (now wife) was pulling the sheets off the bed and made a remark about how much hair was on my pillowcase. I guess it's normal to lose hair while you sleep, but this was enough that she noticed and commented on it. She said it was no big deal – she's always been supportive no matter what, but I decided to look into doing something about it right then. Even though my family had a strong history of male baldness, I didn't know what if anything my relatives had ever done or tried anything for hair loss. No one really talks about it. As I started searching on the internet, I learned that there were a lot of people especially guys my age dealing with it. Once I started seeing it, hair was constantly on my mind and everywhere I went I noticed who had hair, who was losing hair and I was surprised that even I hadn't noticed some of my friends who were losing their hair. Maybe people hadn't noticed it about me either.

I was surprised at how my hair loss made me feel. My girlfriend became my wife and I know she loves me hair or no hair, but for myself – for my own confidence – I decided I wanted to do something about it if I could. I started doing Rogaine. It was easy and I think it helped but I was still losing hair so I visited a hair doctor who prescribed finasteride. I've been on that now for almost 3 years and it's really helped me stabilize the

situation – I'm not really losing any more hair now. The main drawback is that we are thinking about having kids now so I am as careful as I can be about cutting
my finasteride tablet – I don't even let her stay in the same room to be sure that she doesn't come in contact with any dust from the pill. That's a big part of the reason that we ultimately decided to do the SmartGraft hair transplant with Dr. Toyos – I'd rather have a permanent solution and maybe not have to worry about taking medicine for the rest of my life plus I had investigated other transplants techniques before SmartGraft. We wanted the SmartGraft because there were no scars afterward - I didn't want a big scar on the back of my head. After 3 months, the hair that was implanted had fallen out like they told me it would, but then two weeks later, it really started growing back in and my friends started commenting because they noticed how much my hair was beginning to fill in. After that, every week it has looked twice as thick as it did the week before. I used to feel like I looked 10 years older than I am, but I don't feel that way anymore. It has given me my confidence back.

Oral Medications: That Sounds Scary, What Should I Believe?

There are two oral medications that are commonly used for hair regrowth, both of them originally used for other medical purposes and later found to be helpful for growing hair.

The first is finasteride, also known as Propecia and it is a medication that you probably have heard of before. Originally used in men in much higher doses for prostate enlargement, it is the only FDA approved oral medication for hair regrowth and has been on the market for hair since 1997.[30] The second is spironolactone - also known as Aldactone – and it is used mostly for relief of fluid buildup in heart failure or kidney disease but can beis also commonly used for hypertension and low blood potassium unresponsive to other therapies. It also has some hormonal effects that we will discuss later.

First, there are a couple of interesting caveats to know about finasteride. The older version of this medicine, finasteride (also known as Proscar), is available generically in the 5 mg dose and has been since 1992. Only the 1 mg is used in the newer version approved for hair preservation. Because the pharmaceutical world can sometimes be a little upside down, would you believe that the 1 mg is typically much more expensive than the 5 mg? Doesn't make any sense, but it's true so most hair doctors including myself typically recommend that patients purchase the less expensive option and use a pill splitter or other device to break the capsule in half to help patients save some money along with their hair.

The way finasteride works is by blocking the conversion of testosterone to dihydrotestosterone (DHT) which is no friend to hair follicles and primarily responsible for male and female pattern baldness. It specifically inhibits the type 2 5-alpha-reductase enzyme present in high concentrations in and around the hair follicles of balding men.

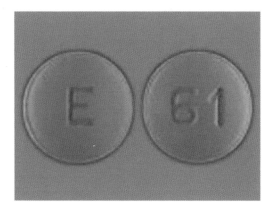

Finasteride suppresses enzymes that are likely responsible for hair follicle death and also helps to restore miniaturized hair follicles to their larger, normal state and the numbers are impressive: after 5 years, 90% of men taking finasteride maintained their hair or increased hair growth with only 10% having lost hair compared to baseline. In contrast, only 6% of men using the placebo had an increase in hair growth and the great majority, 75%, lost hair compared to baseline.[31]

An actual Hair Count Study has been done, hair counts showed an average gain of 277 hairs per square inch at the end of 5 years of finasteride use. The final hairs were significantly larger and heavier than the fine, miniaturized hairs characteristic of balding hair. In the "Hair Weight Clinical Study" 34% improved mean hair mass/ weight difference were observed in the Propecia treatment group.[32] If you decide to use finasteride in your fight against hair loss, the odds are absolutely in your favor. The great majority of people who try it are going to notice that they are keeping their hair, that the number of hairs will increase and that the new hairs that grow in will be larger, thicker and more substantial than the older hairs.

Finasteride results baseline, then every 6 months until the final bottom right photo at 2 years.

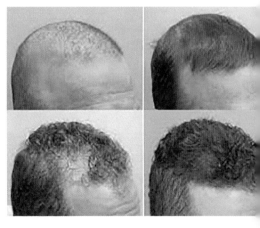

The long-term benefits and adverse events are not known. We do know that the effect of finasteride peaks between 1-2 years, it continues to be effective for at least 5 years. That is as far out as the studies have measured. Finasteride, like a lot of other hair growth products, is what I call a "Cinderella" medicine – you must continue to take it or you return to your normal state. It should be taken once daily with or without meals. It is important to take finasteride continuously for at least one year before you and your doctor can assess whether it is working or not for you. Do not expect results with this medicine in a week or two. It definitely takes some time to build but the results are unparalleled in my opinion.

The sexual side effects of Propecia are where the conversation gets a little more serious. In general, side effects from the low dose are uncommon. At the higher doses – which would include the 5 mg tablet, men (if they are taking 5 mg/day for prostate issues) do face an increased risk in breast cancer. The potential sexual side effects have gotten quite a bit of press because of reports of sexual dysfunction including reduced libido (0.3%), erectile dysfunction (0.3%) and decreased volume of sperm (0.3%). Orgasm disorders have also been reported in both men and women. In most cases, these side effects resolved spontaneously with the discontinuation of the medication but in a select few, side effects have persisted and are known as "post-finasteride syndrome." Because this happens so rarely, there is no clear answer on whether this is psychological, related to the drug or both.

It is true that male fertility may be adversely affected with or without poor semen quality that normalizes or improves after medication discontinuation. The sexual side effects related to finasteride have been reported, but it hasn't been definitively linked as a cause links by studies. Sexual dysfunction is a complex problem and can be caused by a variety of factors. In large scale studies, 3.8% of finasteride users experienced sexual side effects and 2.1% of men receiving placebo reported similar side effects, which turns out to be fairly close.[33] The problem of having the question of sexual dysfunction in your mine is that it can become the elephant in the room. Try NOT to think it and it becomes all you can think about. In some cases, the sexual function could become a self-fulfilling prophecy. When making a decision about usage of finasteride, users should be aware of the risk, aware of the research data and ultimately make the best decision for themselves together with their doctors.

It is also VERY important to note that Propecia should never be used by, near or around pregnant women as the medication can cause birth defects in male children. I caution patients to not even let pregnant or potentially pregnant women come in contact with the medication dust from breaking tablets – it's that serious. Propecia is not officially indicated for women although it is used commonly in post-menopausal women, it is typically not used in women of childbearing potential. Finasteride should not be used in children or those with liver impairment as the drug may not be easily cleared from their bodies.[34]

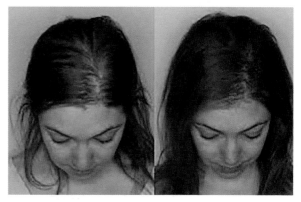

Other less common side effects of Propecia have included reports of skin rash, swelling of lips and face, testicular pain, mood changes including depression and cognitive changes described as "brain fog." These symptoms are significantly less likely to occur (less than 1% chance) but anyone considering it should be aware and fully informed.[35]

SPIRONOLACTONE

This medication is not nearly as controversial in the press. It was discovered in 1957 and is listed in the World Health Organization's List of Essential Medicine as one of the safest and most effective medicines needed for health systems. It was originally used as a diuretic and to lower high blood pressure and later found to have utility in low blood potassium situations unresponsive to oral supplementation. More importantly for our purposes, spironolactone also blocks the effects of testosterone and androgen and has some estrogen like effects. This makes it medically useful for boys experiencing early puberty, women experiencing uncontrolled acne or oiliness and lastly, is part of the treatment cocktail in general reassignment surgeries in transgender women. Unlike finasteride, it can be used safely in pre-menopausal women. Spironolactone is not generally recommended for use in men due to the high risk of feminization (development of breasts, etc) and other side effects unless it is for a short-term acute situation like heart failure.[36]

Low doses of the medication 25-75 mg have been used to stabilize hair loss but higher doses of up to 200 mg can sometimes be more useful. Side effects are generally dose related and can include irregular menses, breast tenderness or enlargement, dry mouth, stomach cramps, diarrhea, headache, dizziness. Like finasteride, spironolactone can also cause a loss of libido. Most importantly, this medication should also be avoided by anyone who may become pregnant because it also causes birth defects. Another common side effect due to the estrogen-like activity is breast tenderness and enlargement.

Because spironolactone is potassium sparing, potassium levels can also rise to dangerous levels (usually without symptoms) and should be checked periodically by your primary care provider while taking this medication.[37] With this warning, I should say that I've seen literally hundreds of young women on this medication, generally for acne, and probably because it is only a very mild diuretic, I've never seen anyone get dehydrated or have an issue with potassium. Many of the patients that have taken it are NFL cheerleaders, exercising nonstop and out on in the field in the heat. Not one of them has every reported an issue with it, but I've always passed along my concern. So, if you decide that taking spironolactone is right for you, drink extra water and get your potassium checked. All in all it has been a reasonably safe drug for people to use for a variety of cosmetic purposes. Also, avoid potassium supplementation, as that can lead to a dangerous buildup of potassium which can cause heart arrhythmias. Finally, I should also warn you that the medication itself has a very distinctive smell, like a skunk or reminiscent of weed, depending on your point of view but it doesn't cause any untoward odors on your body.

Cost: finasteride   average cost is 25-30 dollars/ month
        spironolactone: average cost 30 dollars per month

Growth Factors and PRP

PRP, or platelet rich plasma, has been popular since Kobe Bryant swore to the public and the NBA that PRP injections into his aging knees was the best thing going. Since then, a multitude of A list sports stars needing joint repair have made their way to the same orthopedic clinic in Germany that ultimately made PRP a household term. Tiger Woods made his way over there a few times, A-Rod, and Peyton Manning were just a few of the celebrity athletes that became fans of PRP.

Why did they go? Dr. Peter Wehling, a German orthopedist, first developed the treatment known as Regenokine. Regenokine is regenerative medicine technique that has become a new buzzword in medicine. Regenerative medicine attempts to harness and concentrate the body's ability to heal itself. PRP is just one part of the regenerative medicine movement. Other concentrated or purified growth factors, amniotic membranes, stem cells (Madonna is a fan) are also being used to recreate youthful appearances and function, speed healing and reduce injury.

PRP specifically calls for drawing a certain amount of blood from the patient's body, then spinning it down in a special centrifuge and taking the concentrated natural healing factors off the top of the centrifuged mix (the red blood cells are heavier and sink to the bottom of the container during the centrifuge process). Platelets, as it turns out, a plentiful in growth factors. They contain roughly 30 different kinds of growth factors, many of which are already used extensively in aesthetics to boost the production of hair and collagen, either alone or in conjunction with other procedures. Once the PRP is created, it is removed from the centrifuge for injection or topical application to speed healing or reduce inflammation to a target site. The original formulation called for a slight heating of mixture to simulate the increased cytokine activity of a fever, although the heating is no longer felt to be necessary.[38]

PRP has been in use for many years either as a standalone therapy or combined with microneedling or laser procedures to enhance collagen production and reduce healing time. After Kobe, Kim Kardashian is probably most responsible for putting PRP on the map with the famous Instagram picture of her "Vampire Facial, a patented process that combined microneedling with PRP to amplify the collagen boosting benefits."[39]

We've been using PRP at Toyos Clinic for aesthetics, for dry eye and for hair growth. Here's how it works if a patient decides they want to move forward with PRP for hair growth. I encourage them to come to clinic for their PRP appointment fully hydrated to make the blood

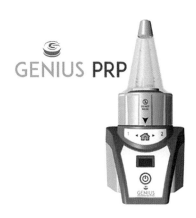

GENIUS PRP

drawing process as fast and easy as possible and I'll offer a bottle of water while they are waiting. The patient gets a small butterfly IV and approximately 60 ccs of blood is removed, spun down in the office and then re-injected fresh into the thinning areas of the scalp. In this way, platelets can be concentrated by a factor of 5-10 compared with untreated blood. Some PRP manufacturers require that the blood is shipped off and returns to the clinic days or weeks later. In fact, for the German clinic, athletes had blood taken at a specific location in the US then specially packaged and shipped to the German clinic for processing. I prefer making PRP on the spot because it seems intuitive to me that doing so would help to preserve and deliver the best results before the product ages or is subject to much jostling or temperature fluctuations but I have not reviewed comparison data. In general, results from PRP take about 3 months to work. The main appeal is that is a natural way to boost your own hair production capture and utilize your body's own growth enhancers.

The exact way PRP works to boost hair growth still isn't entirely clear, but according to some studies it seems to be by a combination of growth factors stimulating the development of new hair follicles as well as the vascular growth factors increasing the circulation and vascularization of the follicle to bring more nutrition to the area. Like Rogaine and cyclosporine, the PRP seems to prolong the growth phase of hair and turn off signals designed to kill the hair follicle prematurely. It may also speed up the resting phase pushing it into actively growing phase of the hair to some degree like prostaglandin activity.[40]

According to some studies, PRP starts working within 10 minutes of injection, with more than 95% of growth factors kicking in within 1 hour. Platelet growth factor synthesis continues to be effective for at least 7 days. [41]The biggest differences between varying preparations of PRP is how much of the patient's original blood is taken and how it is prepared. Depending on the machine, you could end up with platelet poor or platelet rich plasma, and a variable amount of red blood cells and white blood cells. Traditional centrifuges alone produce platelet poor plasma, not particularly helpful for hair growth or collagen boosting and not even worth the needle stick, in my opinion. The Magellan PRP used by orthopedists in the US and in our clinic is about the size and shape of a margarita mixer. It is a no-touch process that is self-contained after the initial blood draw. In less than 5 minutes, your PRP is made and ready to go.

The research studies which have reported hair growth show that most people notice an improvement after about 90 days and offer protocols where patients receive regular injections every 2-4 weeks. Many patients can't afford that or can't commit to monthly clinic visits. For us, I recommend getting all of the PRP injected at once and letting it do its job. If you're getting stuck every few weeks, your scalp is going to end up as sore as your pocketbook.

Overall, PRP is great to have in the armamentarium for hair loss. It boosts hair growth using your body's own growth machinery for those who prefer natural hair regrowth treatments. One notable thing it doesn't do is to address the hormonal component of hair loss. This means PRP a great standalone treatment for younger patients, someone who just had a baby or other hormonal disruption and a great adjunct with hormonal treatment for almost everyone else in addition to the standards of treatment.

Cost: 500-2000 dollars for up to 3 month supply

Low Level Laser Therapy Devices: Caps and Combs

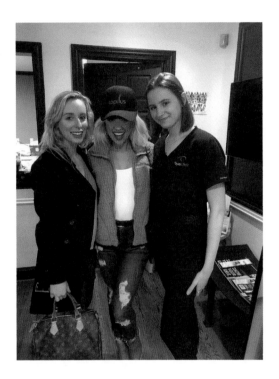

Most of these devices are made to look like low key baseball hats but they come as actual helmets, combs, bonnets, headbands, you name it. Devices like these utilize visible and infrared red light including low level lasers in wavelengths good for jumpstarting the hair follicles by targeting the energy stores there in the range of

600-700 nanometers within the visible light spectrum. The idea is this: using light energy to excite, turn on or restart cells and cellular activity in the hair follicles and scalp that may normally be suppressed due to inflammation or just getting quiet due to normal aging processes. This process is called photobiomodulation or photobiostimulation.

These devices also generate a small amount of heat which may in turn trigger subclinical heat shock proteins in addition to the photobiomodulation processes, that turn on natural reparative and restorative cycles within the follicle. Low level laser lights improve circulation in and around the hair follicles, reduce further hair loss, reverse the miniaturization of hair, increase the density of hair, decrease inflammation, and are even known to modulate the testosterone conversion like finasteride.[42]

The benefits of non-thermal low level laser therapy or LLLT were discovered accidentally in 1967 by Endre Meser, who set out to prove that LLLT was a source of cancer. Imagine his surprise when the lasers proved not only to NOT to be carcinogenic, but instead the mice that he had shaved starting growing dense, thick hair on their backs.[43] Since then, research has been done in a variety of clinical areas showing that low level light is useful for wound healing, wound healing in dental procedures, facial rejuvenation and even for pain relief.

It is true that these devices work equally well for hair loss in both men and women. Some researchers believe that for this light stimulation to work you must have a follicle in place that has the potential to become activated so that Mr. Clean type bald guys or patients with scarred follicles may not respond in a satisfactory way to the energy. However, there is no way to clinically tell the difference between "quiet" and "gone." Just like some batteries are dead and others are "really dead" there is data to suggest the LLLT devices can work even post chemo and in alopecia areata, arguably two of the toughest hair loss situations that exist. We have seen this with meibomian glands in dry eye disease in our own clinic. Glands appear "dead" but are revived with reduction of inflammation or over time with the right amount of energy. I suspect that some follicles may be dying, others chronically inflamed, or just slowing down with age. I don't believe in writing off any situations before we try it to see what might happen, just in case we are pleasantly surprised. More follicles than we may necessarily suspect have the potential to respond favorably to the influx of energy to jump start them.

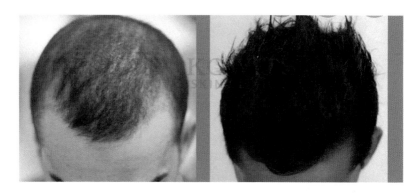

Like PRP, using low level light can be perceived as a more "natural" approach without the side effects of medications. Like Rogaine and finasteride, low level light therapy for hair loss was approved in 2007 by the FDA and the devices themselves are generally cleared by the FDA.

When you google low level light hair device, and literally hundreds of options pop up. How can you choose the best light for you? There are two main distinctions between devices. 1. The number of diodes or energy generating devices and 2. The quality of the light. Many of the devices out on the internet are cheaply made and minimally effective, if at all. You can really spend a lot of money on what is basically junk. Stuff that isn't going to work well or will take so long that you'll grow tired of it and toss it before you see results. Knowing the basic principles will help when you go shopping for hair caps. The first principle is, the more diodes the better. You will see best results with more diodes – at least 272 and preferably 312 diodes like the CapillusRX, physician strength and available only through physician's offices. Plenty of devices out there have a smaller number of diodes: 80 diodes, 120 that are primarily just homeopathic doses of energy – useful for only the mildest hair loss, if at all. There is a reason that the CapillusRx hat is only available through an MD and that is because it is head and shoulders more effective than the others on the market. Physician strength, if you will. Having this level of energy is the difference between having to wear a hat 30 minutes per day versus wearing the CapillusRX 6 minutes per day plus seeing more results faster. One of the best things about the cap is that there are virtually no known adverse side effects although some patients have reported minor scalp itching from the small amount of heat generated. I personally like to offset the small amount of heat and potential drying of the scalp with the small amount of Vitamin A included in the Rogaine Plus mixture.

What should you expect? In the first 3 months of use, most of my patients start to notice a reduction in shedding of hair. Some patients can see a temporary increase in shedding as hair follicles get synced in the growth phase. The company advises that an increased density of hair for the average patients should start at the 3-6 month mark. At the one-year mark, thicker fuller hair should be noticeably apparent and peak results are noticed at 2 years.[44] One study noted an average increase of 17 hairs per square centimeter after usage for just 6 months.[45]

Low level laser therapy is different from the "more is better" theories of hair growth. Certainly, more low-level lasers seem to be helpful from a growth standpoint, but too much of a good thing (more than 5mW/cm squared) can actually be damaging to growing hairs. There are still questions that remain as to the ideal amount of energy needed, how different skin types/hair color may or may not affect the absorption, the best candidates for hair growth with low level lasers, and the ideal wavelength or range of wavelengths.[46]

Many people choose the hair cap light option because it's neat, it's fast, it works and it has little to no side effects, unlike some of the other FDA approved hair growth options. Just like other hair treatments, it takes time and it's important to choose the best technology for optimal hair growth and stick with it for best results. There is also data to suggest that red light works synergistically with other hair boosting products like Rogaine and hair transplant, amplifying the effects.[47] In transplant, LLLT reduces inflammation and improves wound healing, so that patients undergoing transplant are counseled to for the short term postoperative period to use it to speed healing and to ensure viability of transplants. Long term, the LLLT cap helps to maintain the viability of the transplants, boosts their growth and helps to maximize results. More studies are needed to help us understand all that this treatment modality has to offer.[48]

Cost: from 60/single session with cap in office – 3500 for personal cap for daily at home use

Steve's story

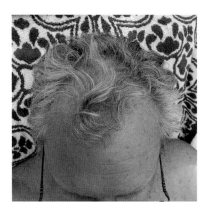

My story is going to be a little bit different. I started going bald in my 40's but didn't really think much of it because it was mostly hidden by a big tuft of hair in the front. It wasn't really a big deal to me, my friends and family joked about it but I just chalked it up to getting older. I sort of looked into treatments for it but nothing really appealed to me. I didn't really want to spend the money, the time or the effort to do something every day and I looked into hair transplant surgery but it was really out of the questions – too much risk, too much down time, too expensive for something that wasn't much of a problem in my opinion. Plus, my wife loves me so what do I care?

For me, the hair loss wasn't in a traditional pattern, I kept a patch in front and literally lost a U-shaped area of hair behind it – like an island in the front. I'm not really bald and I don't really have a full head of hair – kind of in between. The rest of my hair was pretty good though, thick enough, and it grows fast enough for me to need a haircut about every 2 weeks. It was really my wife who suggested getting SmartGraft. One day at the pool, she was standing over me and said something about the spot getting bigger. She did all the research and decided that SmartGraft was the way to go mainly because of the success rate of the grafts and because it didn't leave a big scar the way older procedures did.

So that's how I found myself getting a consult for hair transplantation surgery. I met with Dr. Toyos and we decided that about 500 grafts would be perfect for filling in the area behind my "island." I don't remember much from the grafting part, I think I pretty much slept through the whole thing. I remember waking up to go to the bathroom, we got some lunch and I watched shows on my phone while they were working on placing the grafts in the afternoon. For me, the post op instruction were pretty straightforward, not too difficult and didn't take up much time. You basically just have to be gentle with the grafts, not too rough and everything will go fine. We were careful not to get direct shower spray on the grafts in the shower and I spent about a week with button up shirts so that I didn't traumatize the grafts by pulling my shirt over my head. I did wear a hat though because I got my grafts in summer and I like to be outside. You should wear a hat to protect against the sun, just not too tight right after the transplant.

 I know that I could do more things to maximize my hair like using topical medicines, taking pills or buying the light cap and I might one day. I might ask for the cap for Christmas, now that I think about it! But at the end of the day, I know myself and I like to keep things simple. The grafts have been really all I think I need right now and I'm really happy about how good they are starting to look after 6 months!

Surgical Options: No More Linear Scars

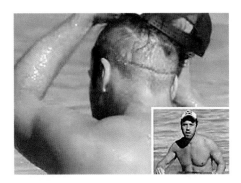

Every so often the pictures would appear. Celebrities letting down their guard and jumping into the ocean to have a little summer fun. That's when the paparazzi would take advantage of the situation and jump in with a close up zoom photos of the telltale linear white scar on the back of their heads that told their celebrity secrets: they'd undergone hair transplants.

The scars themselves were bad enough. Not only did you have to worry about your tea getting spilled when your hair got wet (for men) but men also were forever doomed to never again wearing their hair short. Fashionable fades are not possible for you with big thick ropy scars back there. Which brings me to the real reason that this eye surgeon got into hair: because now we have technology that is precise, elegant and light years better than what we had even ten years ago. SmartGraft Follicular Unit Extraction (a fancy way of saying that we are removing hairs 1 and 2 at a time).

The extraction piece is a small, circular suction powered device that cores out a single follicular unit at a time. This unit is sucked through the system and lands in one of two refrigerated canister holding units which are sprayed with chilled saline or chilled growth solution at regular intervals. The cooled follicular units can be collected until the canister is full without sacrificing any of the viability of the grafts, making the harvesting process more streamlined. Once the canisters are full, the units can be placed on chilled petri plates and kept until time to insert the grafts. The process still takes time but is dramatically more efficient with this technology. You can precisely remove and implant the hair one and two follicles at a time in a way that is slightly reminiscent of the elegance of eye surgery.

In the bad old days, a big huge chunk of scalp (think 3 inches by 5 inches or more) was literally cut from the back of your head and then dissected into a few follicles at a time to be implanted. That left you with the dreaded white scar of shame and depending on how OCD your surgeon was, a possibility for the doll like chunky implants of yesterday to sprout unattractively on your head. Plus, the massive head wound in the back made it was a week or two before you could sleep on your back if you were so inclined. The worst part, in my mind, was that hair loss was already embarrassing and sometimes shameful to the people that were suffering. With the stripmethod, there was so much obvious physical evidence to show what you had done, it was almost impossible to receive a undercover hair transplant without practically announcing your secret from the rooftops.

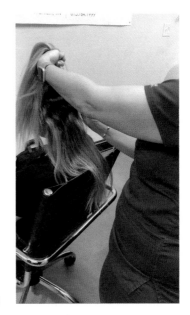

All of that changed with the advent of the SmartGraft machine. The SmartGraft machine made it possible to separate the hairs a few follicles at a time, to remove them easily, to store them in a way that preserves their viability, to streamline the transplantation process and implant hair follicles with a high degree of success given their unique system.

First, just like the strip method, hair is generally harvested from what I call the "Forever Hair" zone which is the strip of hair on the backside of your head between your eyes that also happens to be DHT (the testosterone derivative) resistant. Whatever else happens, genetically or hormonally to you, this hair is forever hair. Take a look at my husband if you'd like a better illustration of this. The hair he has left is Forever Hair (which is fine – I like him just the way he is). When we implant this hair, it becomes Forever Hair at the new site. It is not affected by genetics or hormones in the way that the hair that was originally there was or will be. If you happen to be running low in the scalp hair department, other body hair can also be used in the transplant process if needed, including chest, back and beard hair. Some men have more body hair than scalp hair so this is primarily the situations in which we would consider using body hair for transplant because it tends to be coarser than scalp hair.

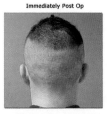
Immediately Post Op

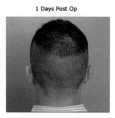
1 Days Post Op

Follicular Unit Extraction Donor Healing

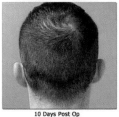
10 Days Post Op

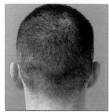
3 Weeks Post Op

When you decide to have SmartGraft, there are a few things you will need to do to prepare for the procedure. First, you can either get a close cut at your normal hairdresser's or we can do it on the day of the procedure. Women have it a little easier because their overlying hair naturally covers the operative site. For guys, it will probably surprise you as much as it did me to learn that it only takes about a week for the graft site on the head to heal so that it is not noticeable to others. If you color your hair, go ahead and touch up your roots right before the transplant. We have to wait 8 weeks after transplant to color which can be plenty enough time for the "glitter" in your hair to start showing so you might as well get yourself a head start beforehand.

Discontinue any prescription or over the counter blood thinners (coumadin, heparin, garlic, ginseng, ginkgo, vitamin E or fish oil) starting 2 weeks before the procedure with the prescribing doctor's okay. It's also important to avoid alcohol for at least 48 hours before the surgery. Plan to wear comfortable clothes to the procedure especially a button-down shirt, zippered or wide-necked pullover that will be easy to get over your head and won't tug or pull on the surgical site or the new grafts. Don't bring a shirt that you are very attached to, sometimes a little blood can find its way onto a shirt. (Cold water is helpful for getting it out.) Bring a shirt that is okay to get soiled and one you can live without if necessary. Get a good night's sleep and be sure to eat a good breakfast before coming in for the procedure. The relaxing medicine can irritate your stomach, so you'll want to take it with food in your stomach to avoid stomach upset.

If you have any medication allergies, be sure to let your doctor know. If your appointment is in the afternoon, a light lunch is fine. Smokers never heal as well as non-smokers, so if you are able, quit or cutdown at least 2 weeks prior to the procedure and for 8 weeks afterwards. You can do it! Patients with certain medical conditions may need medical clearance in order to proceed, this should be taken care of at least 3 weeks prior to the scheduled procedure.

The night before, it is good to wash your face, scalp and neck with an antibacterial soap or a disinfecting spray that is appropriate for the face. We prefer Avenova, a hypochlorous solution that kills bacteria and viruses and is even safe enough to use around the delicate eye area. If you wear a hairpiece, hair system or extensions, make sure they are removed prior to your shower the night before surgery and not replaced as they can carry bacteria that could cause infection in the surgery sites. All glue products should be removed from your hair and scalp prior to the procedure. If you want to wear a certain hat or hats after the procedure, bring it or them into the office so we will assess and adjust the fit and give instructions on how to put it on and take it off.

From a surgical standpoint, prior to your procedure, an evaluation of your medical history, medication history, prior surgeries and expectation will be covered. Photographs of every angle of your head will be taken. Your scalp will be examined to determine hair density, the potential number of grafts that can reasonably be taken, to look for any potential problems and to determine the right number of grafts for your goals. Again, hair is generally taken from the Forever Hair Zone but body and beard hair can also be transplanted. It is not

possible to "donate" hair follicles to a friend although it might work between identical twins. Most people receive anywhere from 500 to 2,000 grafts in a session. Five hundred is typical for eyebrows and supplementing small frontal areas. Two thousand grafts will cover an area roughly the size of a CD (remember those?) although we can stretch the amount of territory we cover by blending and feathering some of the grafts.

Your doctor will outline the area for transplantation, staggering the front line of the hair for a natural appearance and taking into consideration potential for further hair loss on the sides or

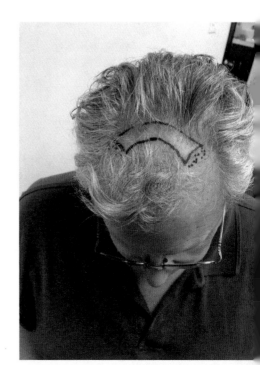

the crown. You want to be sure that your transplanted hair "fits" and continues to look natural even as you age if the worst happens an more hair is naturally lost due to genetics or hormones.

Five hundred grafts will take the morning or the afternoon and two thousand is an all day affair. One of the many benefits of SmartGraft is the ability to perform the procedure in the office and not to have to schedule operating room or surgery center time. I have patients bring in headphones and whatever they like for entertainment (as long as the content is suitable for everyone, please) and plan for them to have a driver pick them up after the procedure. I offer relaxing medicine so many people sleep through the majority or all of the process. The first part of the procedure – usually the morning- is spent face down on your stomach getting the topical numbing medicine and then harvesting the grafts.

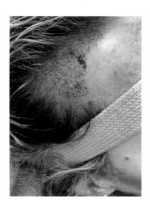

The SmartGraft machine is special because it uses suction assist harvesting to gently and precisely extract follicular units (or hair). The machine keeps count automatically It also cools and sprays the grafts intermittently to keep them moist and viable. This is the part of the process where a lot of viable grafts were lost with previous hair harvesting methods because hair requires nutrition and too much time away from a good blood supply or exposure to room temperature meant grafts were lost or DOA upon transplant. This upgrade in technology has resulted in graft viability of upwards of 95%, which helps to guarantee the result you are looking for.

Once the right number of grafts have been collected, patients generally have a little lunch and are turned over and able to sit up for the graft placement. Patients are able to pop into the restroom anytime they need to during the day. The grafts that have been harvested are examined to make sure they are suitable (not transected or cut at the root) and the implantation process begins. There are several ways to make the incision with a needle or with a scalpel but making a tiny, self-sealing incision that hugs and grabs the implant is the best and fastest way to get them acclimated to their new home. Because we take the hairs one and two at a time, once healing is complete is no linear scar on the back of the head and the small holes made on the front and the back of the scalp during the procedure close up rapidly due to the high degree of vascularization in the scalp.

After the procedure a few things to remember: no alcohol for at least 48 hours, Tylenol and Advil are generally sufficient for pain and your doctor may write a prescription for something a little stronger. You should sleep upright preferably in a recliner the first night to help with scab formation and reduce swelling. An ice pack to the eyebrows/forehead (20 minutes on and 20 minutes off) will also help reduce forehead swelling the first few days after transplant. Be careful not to put ice directly on the grafts as this may compromise their survival. It can be normal to experience a little bit of bleeding from the incision sites the first night or two. You will want to cover your pillow with a towel for the first few nights.If the bleeding persists or you are unable to control it with mild pressure, contact your doctor. Scabs will naturally form within a few hours of the pressure and will fall off when sufficient healing has occurred generally within 1-2 weeks. Itching means healing but resist the urge to scratch or lift scabs anywhere in the graft region as you can damage the grafts. No hair washing for at least 24 hours and when you do get back in to wash your hair use either a cup to pour water over your head or use a strainer between you and the shower spray to avoid the direct pressure of spray on the new grafts. Never use peroxide on grafts (or any healing area, actually) because it damages more tissue than it helps. I know the bubbles are fun and your mother taught you this was okay, but you have to trust me on this one. Don't use Rogaine for 4 weeks after the transplant. Lastly, it's important to avoid direct sunlight. A very loose-fitting hat is appropriate if you are unavoidably heading outdoors and it makes pretty good camo for the procedure as well.

It's important to know here that the actual little piece of hair that is now sticking out of your scalp will fall out from the stress of the journey but that the follicle will remain and live to sprout another day. It takes 3-9 months to start seeing the brand-new little hairs growing but once they do, even your hairdresser won't be able to tell the difference between your transplants and your natural hair.

SmartGraft hair transplantation technology has changed the way I think about hair transplant. What used to be clunky, inefficient, and permanently scarring is now minimally-invasive, done in the office for patient convenience with minimal recovery time and with incredibly natural results – natural looking because you use your own hair and natural appearing hairlines designed for maximal impact making it ideal for men and women for scalp, eyebrows and even beard regrowth. Using this technology to restore hair makes patients look more youthful and feel more confident. I can honestly say that I never get tired of hearing these testimonials from our patients and from seeing the improvements in their lives.

Cost: 5-10 dollars per graft.
Average number of transplants for eyebrows and beards 500 for a total cost of 2500-5000.

Average number of transplant for frontal hairline 1000-2000 for a total cost of 5,000-20,000.
Maximum number of grafts per transplant day: 2000 for a total cost of 10,000-20,000.

Products That Have Been Helpful

Especially for women, noticeably thinning hair can create feelings that are pretty close to panic. All hair regrowth treatments take time, so how best to manage while you need hair solutions today while you are waiting on all your treatments to kick in? I have some pointers from personal experience and ideas I've picked up from others.

Let's start in the shower with shampoos and conditioners. I'm not a big fan of medicated shampoos like Nioxin, the active ingredients aren't super concentrated and the products don't stay in contact with the scalp really long enough to make a difference anyway. If you have dandruff, by all means use a dandruff shampoo - cutting out the chronic inflammation can free your hair up to grow. If you want to use a specific thickening shampoo, I particularly like the new Bumble Thickening line which gently cleanses and volumizes without weighing the hair down otherwise, save your money for things that will make a bigger impact.

Conditioners – for thinning hair, it's important to keep hair moisturized but not to coat it or weigh it hair down. For processed, damaged or post-extension hair, nothing is better to start with than Olaplex products. They have magically built an entire product line out of hair repair chemistry that rebuild broken disulfide bonds in the hair to restore hair and help it continue to grow without breaking. It doesn't volumize, but it will give you an excellent base to heal hair so you can move on to volumizing. And just like the gym, the more you use it, the better your hair gets. Most hair professionals I know use it once a week. The Olaplex product line ranges from daily products to weekly and once a quarter post processing moisturizing treatment. For daily conditioning use, I use the Bumble thickening that uses a silicone smoothing, hydrolyzed proteins for amino acid building and volume along with an ayurvedic component from the gooseberry called amla that is a strong anti-inflammatory and antioxidant and causes the hair shaft to swell and expand.

Out of the Shower but Before Blowdry. The first item on this list is foam mousse – especially for women with longer hairstyles adding a golf ball sized clump of mousse the roots of the front and crown will naturally boost the volume where most women need it most.

Bumble Thickening Go Big Treatment – if you only have thirty bucks or one wish on a desert island, THIS is what you want. Dollar for dollar, you get more bang for your buck than any other product I've tried. Use it by spraying on damp hair before blow drying. There are all kinds of thickening agents including acacia Senegal gum which forms a thickening film on the hair to give it plenty of oomph without a weird or crunchy texture and products that cause the actual hair shaft to swell and expand. Almost like extensions in a bottle.

At the Salon. You can do a few things to amp up your hair strategically. Coloring hair is one strategy. Professionally dyed hair is thicker in diameter and usually shinier too. Dying the hair can take its toll chemically on hair (Olaplex can reverse) but the diameter of each strand is thickened, adding volume to skimpy hair.

Strategic Cuts – Going shorter almost always helps to lessen the pull of gravity on hair adding volume and bounce naturally. Layers will naturally help to add fullness while dropping the weight of longer hair.

Highlights – assuming you have enough hair to do it, add high or lowlights is a great way to add depth and dimension while adding the look of fullness. This works especially well if you are lifting the color of darker hair with a lighter scalp as it helps to reduce the contrast.

Creative Tips for Concealing. Dry shampoo is one of the single best ninja undercover hair-boosting product especially when color is the same as your hair. Using it adds texture and volume to the scalp especially the roots while covering the scalp. Hair pencils designed to cover gray will also work to cover bare scalp areas and eyeshadow will do the trick in a pinch.

Cost: variable depending on the salon.
Thickening shampoo and conditioner 60
Thickening mousse 30
Thickening spray 30
Dry shampoo 36
Hair pencil 26
Olaplex 1-7 approximately 28 per at home piece, additional 50-100 in the salon

My routine:

Over the past year, let's call it the great
Hair Loss Experiment of 2019, I have tried a
variety of products, devices and procedures
to get my hair back. My personal hairdresser
is now referring patients to me after seeing
my scalp and hair improve so dramatically
in a short amount of time. It's always
helpful to talk to others that have been
through difficult times and similar
situations and even better when they can
offer a recipe to follow to hopefully get
similar results. Here is the routine that
worked for me over the past year.

Morning:
My morning starts with a cup of yogurt with
2 scoops of marine collagen powder. I put
my CapillusRX cap on while I'm eating
breakfast and checking out the morning's
headlines and take my vitamins afterward.
I'm currently taking these medications/
supplements for hair:

25 mg Spironolactone
3 HairScience vitamin pills daily
1000 iu vitamin D
1 ml Rogaine Plus with cyclosporine,
prostaglandin and vitamin A

Evening
Another 1 ml Rogaine Plus on the car ride home from work

Monthly
Vitamin B12 shot subcutaneously

Quarterly
PRP or other growth factor injection into my scalp

Total cost:
about 75/month for the vitamins and oral medications
100-200/month for PRP or growth factors
2500-3500 for CapillusRX

It's a little high-maintenance, I admit, but I like to see dramatic results and I like to see them fast. About 2 months into my program, I had been concentrating on one specific problem area in my front hair line. When my youngest daughter looked at it, she said "Mom!! Your hair is coming in LUSH in that spot!" From then on, I wanted LUSH in every spot, so I started treating every part of my scalp not just the one area I had been focused on. One year into the program and I love feeling how much thicker my hair feels when I wash it, when I'm putting in a ponytail and just running my hands through it again.

A Word On PCOS

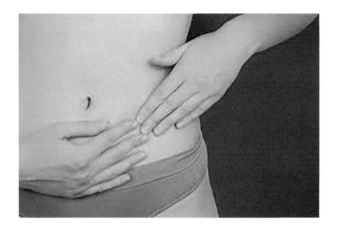

Polycystic Ovary Syndrome (PCO) is a set of symptoms defined by a women's overproduction of androgens. PCO is characterized by irregular or no periods, heavy flow, acne, difficulty getting pregnant, too much hair (hirsutism) or not enough hair. Patients with PCO are also at risk of developing type 2 diabetes, obesity, sleep apnea and endometrial cancers.[49]

PCO is the most common endocrine disorder among women of childbearing age and affects 2-20% of this age group. In a given year, 4 million cases of PCO are reported.[50] It is the most common cause of infertility and may be due to certain environmental agents like bisphenol A, found in many household plastics like water bottles, food storage containers, sports equipment and dvds.

Like so many other situations in hair, it is a mystery why PCO sufferers can have either too much or too little hair. In any case, it is more common that I see those that are suffering from too little hair. The truth is, PCO in large part, is treated just exactly the same as hair loss from aging, genetics or stress with a few important differences.

Metformin is a drug that is commonly prescribed for those suffering with PCO. It is used to treat high levels of blood sugar and insulin in people with diabetes type 2 and those with pre-diabetes. It is currently being studied as a possible anti-aging drug but one of its potential side effects is hair loss. Long term use of metformin is known to reduce the amount of vitamin B12 that is absorbed from your system which may be one of the mechanisms by which hair loss can occur. If you need it, you need it but consider checking levels of B12 and supplementing either orally or with injections if you are low or unsure.

Oral contraceptives or birth control pills are also used to treat PCO. Combining birth control with spironolactone is the most common treatment I see for PCO. The birth control pills suppress ovarian stimulation of the pituitary gland located in the brain and slows the production of androgens in both the ovaries and the adrenal gland.

Some people combine birth control pills with finasteride because finasteride is so effective at reversing hair loss. This combination is a bit of a high wire act in child-bearing women as the finasteride should be stopped at least 6 months prior to attempting conception due to the birth defects that can occur in male fetuses and careful planning is required. Topical minoxidil is commonly recommended either alone or combined together with other therapies.

PCO can be a common and distressing diagnosis for young women dealing with the masculinizing side effects along with acne, obesity, loss of fertility and loss of hair. Hair loss related to PCO can be treated and improved with the right combination of medicines and products.

The Future of Hair Growth

We've come a long way with hair transplants but there's still plenty of opportunities for improvement in the hair growing process. What's next in hair 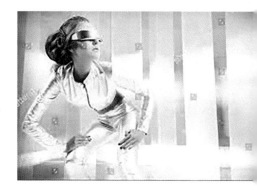 regrowth? One big idea is next generation hair transplants. One of the biggest limiting factors in today's transplant procedures are the limited number of hairs per patient that are available for autografting. Many of the current research is being done to see how that can be improved. One surgeon is looking at transplanting partial hair follicle with only a tiny part of the follicle being used to generate new hair into the recipient area. Using this method could help us stretch the available follicle units and multiply them for better coverage.[51] Along the same idea lines, implanting just a few cells at one time could be another way to stretch out the number of available implants for a given patient. Doctors are also working with the idea of allogeneic grafts – grafts from someone else who could donate follicles for another's use. Up until this point, only identical twins could contemplate the idea of sharing follicles, donations from someone without your exact match would result in rejection of the graft and graft death. The hurdles here are how best to suppress rejection long term and navigating through the legal statutues of the National Organ Transplant Act of 1984 that bans the buying and selling of human organs.[52]

Stem cell transplants using regenerative medicine are another burgeoning idea. The first successful stem cell hair transplant was performed by Italian researchers in 2017.[53] Patients could use stem cells from blood, fat, bone marrow or umbilical or embryonic sources and grow actual hair follicles in the lab. In Asian countries like Japan and Korea, culturally it is less common and also less acceptable for men or women to live with hair loss. This makes it a particularly ripe location for research opportunities. Yokohama National University has been working on this problem for years and now claims to have developed a new way to generate large quantities of stem cells. Although the science may have been printed prematurely, scientists Tokyo's Riken Centre for Developmental Biology are conducting trials to print hair follicles at home and use hair follicles made entirely.[54] In the US, stem cell research and procedures are considered investigational by the FDA. Although they are being performed by some clinics in the US, they are not approved by the FDA and in fact, in 2017, the FDA issued a warning that unapproved stem cell therapies can be harmful and may be illegal and unproven.[55] As of now, there is very little data available on the side effects or success rates of these therapies and no proven techniques yet.

Along with stem cell transplants comes the idea of 3-D printing of hair follicles using live tissue. The idea is to create clones of a person's actual hair then insert them back into the scalp, ideally in overwhelming, unlimited amounts.[56] In a Jetson-type age, a patient could theoretically run their home 3-D printer continuously until the right amount of grafts were made then have a surgeon implant your new head of hair the next day.

What are the hurdles to implementing this technology? One of the main ones has been that once hairs were cloned, they had a tendency to "spread out" within their network and lose the ability to signal one another. Over time, without the signals they needed to stay active, they slowly stopped producing hair. Researchers have recently discovered that if the hair follicle is kept in place by a support structure, a scaffolding, if you will or by using a 3-D printed Jell-O mold type structure for the follicle, the cells can be better kept in place for a better chance at success. Trials are set to begin on some of these ideas within the next year or so by a little company called Allergan, best known for bringing you Botox. It's also worth noting, that these engineered human hair follicles could also be used by researchers to test new types of hair regrowth drugs or treatments.[57]

One idea about attacking hair loss pharmacologically has to do with the idea of completely blocking the hormone DHT. You will remember that arguably the most successful FDA approved medication for hair loss is finasteride or the Propecia which lowers the level of DHT by 65-70% to block the conversion of testosterone. If we could block it entirely or with a more specifically designed molecule, it might be possible to get even better results for even more people with just a tiny little pill every day.[58]

Another pharmacologic agent that may turn out to be useful in the fight against hair loss are a family of drugs that are immunosuppressant and immunomodulators called JAK inhibitors. Part of a family of immunosuppressants known as DMARDS (disease-modifying antirheumatic drugs), these drugs block the binding of some chemical messengers called cytokines to receptors on immune cells that control the production and amplification of even more cytokines that ultimately create more inflammation and damage nearby tissues.[59] They are powerful agents that block what can be called "cytokine storms" and were recently looked at for their utility in blocking the overactive immune reactions that occurred with the COVID-19, Coronavirus also known as SARS-CoV-2.[60] The thought is that by lifting the suppression of inflammation, we can reactivate dormant hair follicles that might have been quieted over time by inflammation and on their way to death.

The interesting thing about using immunomodulators for hair loss like cyclosporine or JAK inhibitors is that the average person, even a bald person has about 100,000 hair follicles on their head. The follicles on the head of a bald person may be dormant or so miniaturized that they only create a tiny, microscopic hair invisible to the naked eye. Usually any hairs that are created with miniaturized follicles have a noticeably different texture, generally described as "wiry." Using immunomodulators or other LLLT/IPL, we can potentially transform these inactive follicles into active ones, the same way IPL can reactivate dormant meibomian glands by theoretically lifting the suppression of inflammation.[61] Sounds great, what could possibly go wrong? The down side of these medicines is that they come along with what are called "black box warnings." Black box warnings are the strongest warning that the FDA can require, showing that the drug in question has been shown by medical studies indicate that the drug carries a significant risk of serious of even life-threatening adverse effects including in the case of JAK inhibitors an increased risk of infections, malignancies and cardiovascular events.[62] Using these medications topically should significantly reduce the risk if not eliminate it outright.

Scientists at Columbia University have recently discovered cells called *trichophages* that likely contribute to our understanding of why immunomodulators have worked in the past to grow hair, even though we didn't understand the mechanism at the time. Their research showed that a previously unseen immune-related cells were found closely associated with resting hair follicles. These cells lurk near inactive follicles and secrete a substance called Oncostatin M that keeps follicles in the dormant state. Blocking these cells with immunomodulators in the lab allowed the hair to restart growth.[63]

From expanding a patient's own available grafts, to allowing for the possibility of donors for hair transplants, to stem cells and 3-D printing to exponentially multiply the number of potential hair grafts, the future of hair regrowth is poised for unprecedented opportunities. I anticipate a day where a single pill daily will stop and reverse hair loss, when people can have all of the transplants they want or need and when new topical agents are available to maximize growth at every stage of hair loss. If you have hair loss issues, they may soon be a part of the hair history.

[1] www.americanhairloss.org accessed March 24, 2020.

[2] Dinh, Q and R Sinclair," Female pattern hair loss: Current Treatment Concepts" Clin Interv Aging 2007 Jun 2(2):189-99.

[3] www.betterhealth.vic.gov.au/Blog/BlogCollectionPage/history-of-hair-loss-treatments, accessed March 25, 2020.

[4] www.history.com/news/9-bizarre-baldness cures, accessed March 25, 2020.

[5] Ibid.

[6] Ibid

[7] www.betterhealth.vic.gov.au/Blog/BlogCollectionPage/history-of-hair-loss-treatments, accessed March 25, 2020.

[8] Ibid.

[9] American Academy of Dermatology "Hair and Scalp Care" accessed March 19, 2020.

[10] Guo, E and R Katta, "Diet and hair loss: effects of nutrient deficiency and supplemental use," Dermatol Pract Concept 2017 Jan;7(1):1-10.

[11] Borowczyk, K, J Suliburska and H Jakubowski, "Demethylation of methionine and keratin damage in human hair" Amino Acids 2018:50(5):537-546.

[12] Sant'Anna Addor F, L Donato, C Melo, "Comparative Evaluation Between Two Nutritional Supplements in the Improvement of Telogen Effluvium," Clin Cosmet Investig Dermtol 2018 Sep 10;11-431-436.

[13] Matsutani, M "Collagen – Skin-Deep in Myth?" Japan Times, Jan 9, 2009.

[14] Kashinath, N, A Garg, P Mithra, and P Manjrekar, "Serum Vitamin D3 levels and Diffuse Hair Fall Among the Studient Population in South India: A Case-Control Study," Int J Trichology 2016 Oct-Dec *(4):160-164.

[15] Patel, D, S Swink, L Castelo-Soccio, " A Review of the Use of Biotin for Hair Loss," Skin Appendage Disord 2017 Aug 3(3):166-169.

[16] Busti, A "Medications Known to Decrease Vitamin B12 Levels," Evidence Based Medicine Consult, www.ebmconsult.com reviewed October 2015 accessed March 28, 2020.

[17] Lucky, A, D Piacquadio, C Ditre, F Dunlap, I Kantor, A Pandya, R Savin, M Tharp,"A Randomized, Placeo-Controlled Trial of 5% and 2% Topical Minoxidil Solutions in the Treatment of Female Pattern Hair Loss" J Am Acad Dermatol 2004 Apr:50(4):541-53.

[18] Suchonwanit P, S Thammarucha, K Leerunyakul, "Minoxidil and Its Use in Hair Disorders: A Review," Drug Des Devel Ther 2019; 13:2777-2786.

[19] Yoo H, Chang I, Pyo H, Kang Y, Lee S, O Kwon, "The Additive Effects of Minoxidil and Retinol on Human Hair Growth in Vitro," Biol Pharm Bull, 2007 Jan:30(1):21-6.

[20] Bazzaro, G, Terezakes N Galen W, Topical Tretinoin for hair growth promotion, J Am Acad Dermatol 1986 Oct; 15(4 Pt 2): 880-3, 890-3.

[21] Shin, H, Won C, Lee S, O Kwon, K Kim, H Eun, "Efficacy of 5% Minoxidil versus Combined 5% Minoxidil and 0.01% Tretinoin for Male Pattern Hair Loss: a Randomized, Double-Blind, Comparative Clinical Trial," Am J Clin Dermtol, 2007, 8(5):285-90.

[22] Barron-Hernandez Y, Tosti A, " Bimatoprost for the Treatment of Eyelash, Eyebrow and Scalp Alopecia," Expert Opin Investig Drugs, 2017 Apr;26(4):515-522.

[23] Gupta A, Mays, R, S Versteen, N Shear, V Piguet, B Piraccini, "Efficacy of Off-Label Topical Treatments for the Management of Androgenetic Alopecia: A Review," Clin Drug Investig, 2019 Mar;39(3):233-239.

[24] El-Ashmayw AA, El-Maadawy, IH, GM El-Maghraby, "Efficacy of Topical Latanoprost versus Minoidil and Betamethasone Valerate on the Treatment of Alopecia Areata.

[25] Takahashi T, A Kamimura " Cyclosporin A Promotes Hair Epithelial Cell Proliferation and Modulates Protein Kinase C Expression and Translocation in Hair Epithelial Cells," J Invest Dermatol 2001 Sept; 117(3):605-11.

[26] Taylor, M A Ashcroft, A Messenger, "Cyclosprin A prolongs human hair growth in vitro," J Invest Dermatol, 1993 Mar; 100(3):237-9.

[27] Buhl, A, D Waldon, M Brunden, "Differences in Activity of Minoxidil and Cyclosporin A on Hair Growth in Nude and Normal Mice. Comparisons of In Vivo and In Vitro Studies," Lab Invest 1990 Jan:62(1):104-7.

[28] Mandal, A, V Gote, D Pal, A Ogundele, A Mitra, "Ocular Pharmacokinetics of a Topical Ophthalmic Nanomicellular Solution of Cyclosporine (Cequa) for Dry Eye Disease," Pharm Res 2019 Jan 7:36(2): 36.

[29] Aldhalm M, N Hadi, F Ghafil, "Promotive Effect of Topical Ketoconazole, Minoxidil, and Minoxidil with Tretinoin on Hair Growth in Male Mice," ISRN Pharmacol 2014 Mar 9, 2014:575423.

[30] "Finasteride Monograph for Professionals" Drugs.com American Society of Health-System Pharmacists. Retrieved 3 April 2020.

[31] Shapiro, J K Kaufman, "Use of Finasteride in the Treatment of Men with Androgenetic Alopecia (Male Pattern Hair Loss), Journal of Investigative Dermatology Symposium Proceedings, Volume 8 Issue 1 June 2003 pp 20-23.

[32] Price,V, E Menefee, M Sanchez, P Ruane,K Kaufman, "Changes in Hair Height and Hair Count in Men with Androgenetic Alopecia after Treatment with Finasteride, 1 mg, daily" J Am Acad Dermatol, 2002 Apr 46(4):517-23.

[33] Mysore, V "Finasteride and sexual side effects" Indian Dermatol Online J 2012 Jan-Apr 3(1):62-65.

[34] Zuuren, E, Z Fedorowicz, J. Schoones, "Interventions for female pattern hair loss," Cochrane Database Syst Rev 2016 May, 2016(5).

[35] Walf, A, S Kaurejo, C Frye, "Research Brief: Self-Reports of a Constellation of Persistent Antiadrogenic, Estrogenic, Physical and Psychological Effects of Finasteride Usage Among Men," Am J Mens Health, 2018 Jul 12(4):900-906.

[36] WebMD, Sprironolactone Oral: Uses, Side Effects, Interactions, Pictures, Warnngs, and Dosing" accessed March 30, 2020.

[37] R Nazarian, A Fairberg, P Hashim, G Goldenberg, "Nonsurgical Hair Restoration Treatment," Cutis, 2019 Jul 104(1):17-24.

[38] Carroll, W " What is This Knee Treatment Kobe Bryant Goes All the Way to Germany For?" www.bleacherreport.com October 4, 2013.

[39] Celletti, E "What Is A Vampire Facial? Everything to Know About the Skin Treatment" Allure, October 26, 2017.

[40] Guo H, W Gao H Endo, K McElwee, "Experimental and Early Investigational Drugs for Androgenetic Alopecia," Expert Opin Investig Drugs, 2017, Aug 26(8):917-932.

[41] Stevens, J S. Khetamal, "Platelet-rich Plasma for Androgenetic Alopecia: A Review of the Literature and Proposed Treatment Protocol," Int J Womens Dermatol 2019 Feb 5(1):46-51.

[42] Panchaprateep, R, T Pisitkum, N. Kalpongnukul, "Quantitative Proteomic Analysis of Dermal Papilla from Male Androgenetic Alopecia Comparing Before and After Treatment with Low Level Laser Therapy," Lasers Surg Med 2019 Sept;51(7):600-608.

[43] Avci, P, G Aurav, J Clark, N Wikonkal, M Hamblin, "Low-Level Laser (Light) Therapy (LLLT) for Treatment of Hair Loss", Lasers Surg Med, 2015 Feb;46(2) 144-151.

[44] CapillusRx website, accessed March 23, 2020.

[45] Suchonwanit, P, N Chalermoj, S Khunkhet, "Low-Level Laser Therapy for the Treatment of Androgenetic Alopecia in Thai Men and Women: A 24-Week, Randomized, Double-Blind, Sham Device Controlled Trial," Lasers in Medical Science, Vol 34: pp1107-1114, 2019.

[46] Suchonwanit, P et al.

[47] Faghihi, G, S Mozafarpoor, A Asilian, F Mokhtari, A Esfahani, B Bafandeh, S Nouaei, M Nilforoushzadeh, S Hosseini, "The Effectiveness of Adding Low-Level Light Therapy to Minoxidil 5% Solution in the Treatment of Patients with Androgenetic Alopecia," Indian J Dermatol Venereol Leprol,, 2018 Sep-Oct;84(5):547-553.

[48] Avci, P et al.

[49] Futterweit, W "A Patient's Guide: Managemnet of Hair Loss in Polycystic Ovary Syndrome," Infertility, Pregnancy and Birth, Polycystic Ovary Syndrome October 11, 2011.

[50] Azziz, R, C Marin, L Hoq, E Badamgarav, P Song, "Health Care-Related Economic Burden of the Polycystic Ovary Syndrome During the Reproductive Life Span, " The Journal of Clinical Endocrinology and Metabolism 90(8)4650-4658.

[51] Cox, D "The New Growth in Hair Loss Research," The Guardian, online Sat 7 2019 accessed March 25, 2020.

[52] "Buying and Selling Organs for Transplantation in the United States: National Organ Transplant Act of 1984 (NOTA) Ban Buying and Selling," Medscape accessed Thursday March 26, 2020.

[53] www.healthline.com/ealth/stem-cell-hair -transplant, accessed March 25, 2020.

[54] Cox, D "The New Growth in Hair Loss Research," The Guardian, online Sat 7 2019 accessed March 25, 2020.

[55] www.fda.gov/consumer-updates/fda-warns-about-stem-cell-therapies, accessed March 25, 2020.

[56] Hamblin, J "Soon There Will Be Unlimited Hair," The Atlantic, July 25, 2019.

[57] Ibid

[58] Hurley, A "The Bald Truth: Everything You Need to Know About Hair Restoration in 2020," Robb Report March 4, 2020.

[59] Columbia University Irving Medical Center, "Studies Uncover New Approaches to Combat Hair Loss in Men and Women," Medical Press News, June 25, 2019.

[60] Stebbing, J, A Phelan, I Griffin, C Tucker, O Oechsle, D Smith, "COVID-19: Combining Antiviral and Anti-inflammatory Treatments," The Lancet Infectious Diseases, February 27, 2020.

[61] Yin Y, Liu N, Gong L, N Song, "Changes in the Meibomian Gland After Exposure to Intense Pulsed Light in Meibomian Gland Dysfunction (MGD) Patients" Curr Eye Res 2018, Mar 43(3):308-313.

[62] www.pfizerpro.com accessed March 26, 2020.

[63] Columbia University Irving Medical Center, "Studies Uncover New Approaches to Combat Hair Loss in Men and Women," Medical Press News, June 25, 2019.